Exercise Steps

Endurance, Strength, Balance, Flexibility

By James Lee Anderson

(ILLUSTRATED)

CONTENTS

EXERCISE: HOW TO GET STARTED

Safety First

Start Out Slowly

Most older adults, regardless of age or condition, will do just fine increasing their physical activity to a moderate level. However, if you haven't been active for a long time, it's important to start out at a low level of effort and work your way up slowly.

When to Check with Your Doctor

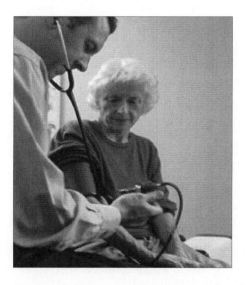

If you are at high risk for any chronic diseases such as heart disease or diabetes, or if you smoke or are obese, you should check first with your doctor before becoming more physically active.

Other reasons to check with your doctor before you exercise include

- Any new, undiagnosed symptom
- Chest pain

- Irregular, rapid, or fluttery heart beat
- Severe shortness of breath

Check with your doctor if you have

- Ongoing, significant, and undiagnosed weight loss
- Infections, like pneumonia, accompanied by fever which can cause rapid heart beat and dehydration
- An acute blood clot
- A hernia that is causing symptoms such as pain and discomfort

Check with your doctor if you have

- Foot or ankle sores that won't heal
- Persistent pain or problems walking after a fall -- you might have a fracture and not know it
- Eye conditions such as bleeding in the retina or a detached retina. Also consult your doctor after a cataract removal or lens implant, or after laser treatment or other eye surgery.

Check with your doctor if you have

- A weakening in the wall of the heart's major outgoing blood vessel called an abdominal aortic aneurysm
- A narrowing of one of the heart's valves called critical aortic stenosis
- Joint swelling.

If You've Had Hip Replacement

If you have had hip repair or replacement

- Check with your doctor before doing lower-body exercises.
- Don't cross your legs.
- Don't bend your hips farther than a 90-degree angle.
- Avoid locking the joints in your legs into a strained position.

Discuss Your Activity Level

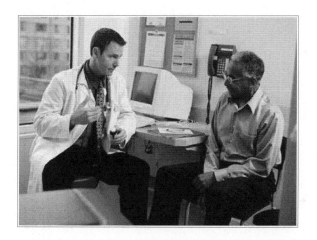

Your activity level is an important topic to discuss with your doctor as part of your ongoing preventive health care. Talk about exercise at least once a year if your health is stable, and more often if your health is getting better or worse over time so that you can adjust your exercise program. Your doctor can help you choose activities that are best for you and reduce any risks.

Tips to Avoid Injury

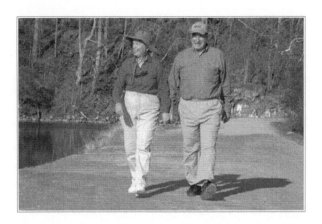

When you exercise, it is important to do it safely. Follow these tips to avoid injury.

- When starting an exercise program, begin slowly with low-intensity exercises.
- Wait at least 2 hours after eating a large meal before doing strenuous exercise.
- Wear appropriate shoes for your activity and comfortable, loose-fitting clothing that allows you to move freely but won't catch on other objects.
- Warm up with low-intensity exercises at the beginning of each exercise session.
- Drink water before, during, and after your exercise session.
- When exercising outdoors, pay attention to your surroundings -- consider possible traffic hazards, the weather, uneven walking surfaces, and strangers.

When to Stop Exercising

Stop exercising if you:

- Have pain or pressure in your chest, neck, shoulder, or arm
- Feel dizzy or sick to your stomach
- Break out in a cold sweat
- Have muscle cramps
- Feel severe pain in joints, feet, ankles, or legs

ENDURANCE EXERCISES

To get all of the benefits of physical activity, try all four types of exercise -- endurance, strength, balance, and flexibility. This section discusses endurance activities.

"Exercise: Enjoyment is Key"

Activities That Increase Breathing and Heart Rate

Endurance exercises are activities that increase your breathing and heart rate for an extended period of time. Examples are walking, jogging, swimming, raking, sweeping, dancing, and playing tennis. Build up your endurance gradually, starting with as little as 5 minutes of endurance activities at a time, if you need to. Then try to build up to at least 30 minutes of moderate-intensity endurance activity on most or all days of the week. Doing less than 10 minutes at a time won't give you the desired heart and lung benefits

Safety Tips

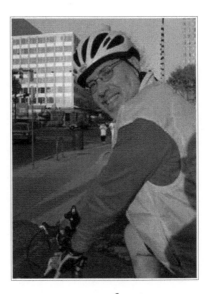

- Do a little light activity, such as easy walking, before and after your endurance activities to warm up and cool down.
- Drink liquids when doing any activity that makes you sweat.
- Dress appropriately for the heat and cold. Dress in layers if you're outdoors so you can add or remove clothes as needed.
- When you're out walking, watch out for low-hanging branches and uneven sidewalks.
- Walk during the day or in well-lit areas at night, and be aware of your surroundings.
- To prevent injuries, use safety equipment such as helmets for biking.
- Endurance activities should not make you breathe so hard that you can't talk and should not cause dizziness or chest pain.

Moderate Endurance Activities to Try

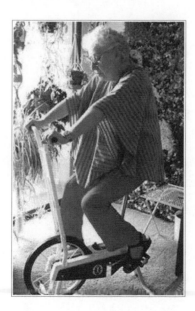

Here are some examples of moderate endurance activities for the average older adult. Older adults who have been inactive for a long time will need to work up to these activities gradually.

- walking briskly on a level surface
- swimming
- dancing
- gardening, mowing, raking
- cycling on a stationary bicycle
- bicycling
- playing tennis

Vigorous Endurance Activities to Try

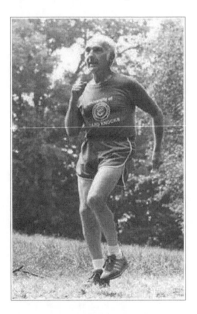

These are examples of activities that are vigorous. People who have been inactive for a long time or who have certain health risks should not start out with these activities.

- playing basketball

8

- jogging
- climbing stairs or hills
- shoveling snow
- brisk bicycling up hills
- digging holes

Work Your Way Up Gradually

Gradually working your way up is especially important if you have been inactive for a long time. It may take months to go from a very long-standing sedentary lifestyle to doing some of the activities suggested in this section.

When you're ready to do more, build up the amount of time you spend doing endurance activities first, then build up the difficulty of your activities. For example, gradually increase your time to 30 minutes over several days to weeks (or even months, depending on your condition) by walking longer distances. Then walk more briskly or up steeper hills.

STRENGTH EXERCISES

Exercises That Build Muscle

Strength exercises build muscle, and even very small changes in muscle strength can make a real difference in your ability to perform everyday activities like carrying groceries, lifting a grandchild, or getting up from a chair.

Strength Exercises to Try

The 10 muscle strengthening exercises which follow include

1. wrist curls
2. arm curls
3. side arm raises
4. elbow extensions
5. chair dips
6. seated rows with resistance band
7. back leg raises
8. knee curls
9. leg straightening exercises
10. toe stands

What to Use, How to Start

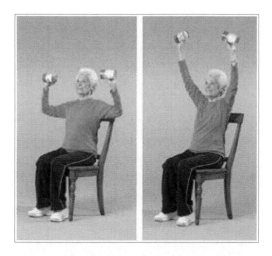

To do most of these strength exercises, you need to lift or push weights. You can use weights, resistance bands, or common objects from your home. Or, you can use the strength-training equipment at a fitness center or gym. Start with light weights and gradually increase the amount of weight you use. Starting out with weights that are too heavy can cause injury. If you can't lift or push a weight 8 times in a row, it's too heavy for you, and you should reduce the amount of weight.

How Much, How Often?

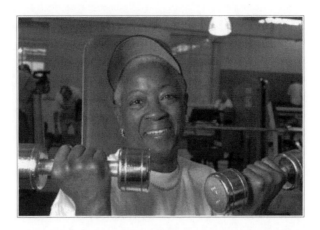

Try to do strength exercises for all of your major muscle groups on 2 or more days per week for 30 minutes at a time, but don't exercise the same muscle group on any 2 days in a row. When using weights, take 3 seconds to lift or push a weight into place, hold the position for 1 second, and take another 3 seconds to return to your starting position. Don't let the weight drop; returning it slowly is very important.

Muscle strength is progressive over time. Gradually increase the amount of weight you use to build strength. When you can do 2 sets of 10 to 15 repetitions easily, increase the amount of weight at your next session.

Safety Tips

- Don't hold your breath during strength exercises. This could affect your blood pressure, especially if you have heart disease.
- Use smooth, steady movements to bring weights into position. Avoid jerking or thrusting movements.

- Breathe out as you lift or push a weight and breathe in as you relax.
- Avoid locking the joints of your arms and legs into a strained position. To straighten your knee, tighten your thigh muscles. This will lift your kneecaps and protect them.
- For exercises that require a chair, choose one that is sturdy and stable enough to support your weight when seated or when holding on during the exercise.

Wrist Curls

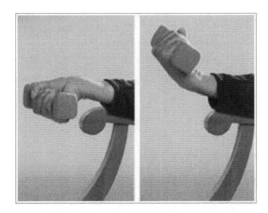

Strengthen your wrists with wrist curls.

1. Rest your forearm on the arm of a sturdy chair with your hand over the edge.
2. Hold weight with palm facing upward.
3. Slowly bend your wrist up and down.
4. Repeat 10 to 15 times.
5. Repeat with other hand 10 to 15 times.
6. Repeat 10 to 15 more times with each hand.

Arm Curls

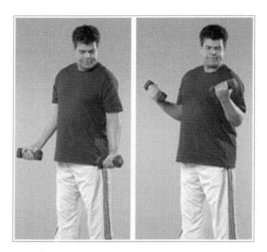

Strengthen your upper arm muscles with arm curls.

1. Stand with your feet shoulder-width apart.
2. Hold weights straight down at your sides, palms facing forward. Breathe in slowly.
3. Breathe out as you slowly bend your elbows and lift weights toward chest. Keep elbows at your sides.
4. Hold the position for 1 second.
5. Breathe in as you slowly lower your arms.
6. Repeat 10 to 15 times.
7. Rest; then repeat 10 to 15 more times.

Side Arm Raises

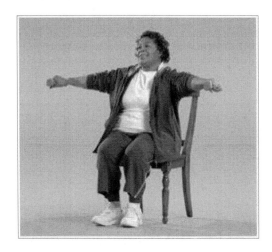

Strengthen your shoulders with side arm raises.

1. You can do this exercise while standing or sitting in a sturdy, armless chair.
2. Keep feet flat on the floor even, shoulder-width apart.
3. Hold hand weights straight down at your sides with palms facing inward.
4. Slowly breathe out as you raise both arms to the side, shoulder height.
5. Hold the position for 1 second.
6. Breathe in as you slowly lower arms to the sides.
7. Repeat 10 to 15 times.
8. Rest; then repeat 10 to 15 more times.

Elbow Extensions

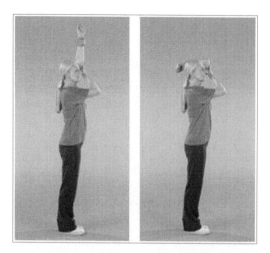

Strengthen the muscles in the back of your arms with elbow extensions.

1. You can do this exercise while standing or sitting in a sturdy, armless chair.
2. Keep your feet flat on the floor, shoulder-width apart.
3. Hold weight in one hand with palm facing inward. Raise that arm toward ceiling.
4. Support this arm below elbow with other hand. Breathe in slowly.
5. Slowly bend raised arm at elbow and bring weight toward shoulder.
6. Hold position for 1 second.
7. Breathe out and slowly straighten your arm over your head. Be careful not to lock your elbow.
8. Repeat 10 to 15 times.
9. Repeat 10 to 15 times with other arm.
10. Repeat 10 to 15 more times with each arm.

Chair Dips

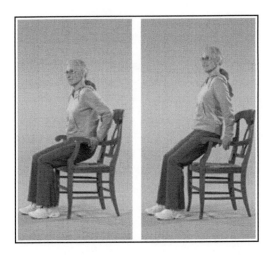

Strengthen your arm muscles with chair dips.

1. Sit in a sturdy chair with armrests with your feet flat on the floor, shoulder-width apart.
2. Lean slightly forward; keep your back and shoulders straight.
3. Grasp arms of chair with your hands next to you. Breathe in slowly.
4. Breathe out and use your arms to push your body slowly off the chair.
5. Hold position for 1 second.
6. Breathe in as you slowly lower yourself back down.
7. Repeat 10 to 15 times.
8. Rest; then repeat 10 to 15 more times.

Seated Row with Resistance Band

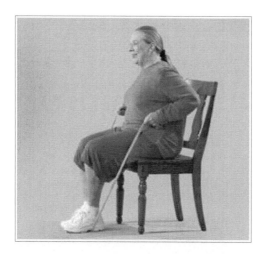

Strengthen your upper back, shoulder, and neck muscles by doing a seated row with a resistance band.

1. Sit in a sturdy, armless chair with your feet flat on the floor, shoulder-width apart.
2. Place the center of the resistance band under both feet. Hold each end of the band with palms facing inward.
3. Relax your shoulders and extend your arms beside your legs. Breathe in slowly.
4. Breathe out slowly and pull both elbows back until your hands are at your hips.
5. Hold position for 1 second.
6. Breathe in as you slowly return your hands to the starting position.
7. Repeat 10 to 15 times.
8. Rest; then repeat 10 to 15 more times.

Back Leg Raises

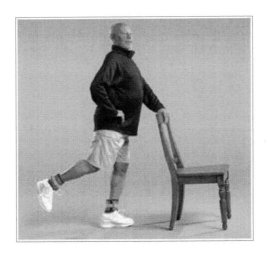

Strengthen your buttocks and lower back with back leg raises.

1. Stand behind a sturdy chair, holding on for balance. Breathe in slowly.
2. Breathe out and slowly lift one leg straight back without bending your knee or pointing your toes. Try not to lean forward. The leg you are standing on should be slightly bent.
3. Hold position for 1 second.
4. Breathe in as you slowly lower your leg.
5. Repeat 10 to 15 times.
6. Repeat 10 to 15 times with other leg.
7. Repeat 10 to 15 more times with each leg.

Knee Curls

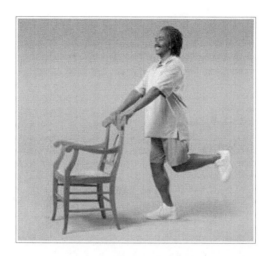

Strengthen muscles in the back of the thigh with knee curls.

1. Stand behind a sturdy chair, holding on for balance. Lift one leg straight back without bending your knee or pointing your toes. Breathe in slowly.
2. Breathe out as you slowly bring your heel up toward your buttocks as far as possible. Bend only from your knee, and keep your hips still. The leg you are standing on should be slightly bent.
3. Hold position for 1 second.
4. Breathe in as you slowly lower your foot to the floor.
5. Repeat 10 to 15 times.
6. Repeat 10 to 15 times with other leg.
7. Repeat 10 to 15 more times with each leg.

Leg Straightening Exercises

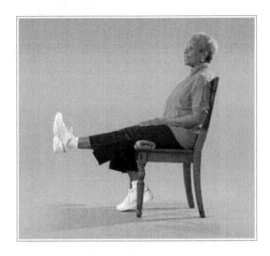

Strengthen your thighs with leg straightening exercises.

1. Sit in a sturdy chair with your back supported by the chair. Only the balls of your feet and your toes should rest on the floor. Put a rolled bath towel at the edge of the chair under thighs for support. Breathe in slowly.
2. Breathe out and slowly extend one leg in front of you as straight as possible, but don't lock your knee.
3. Flex foot to point toes toward the ceiling. Hold position for 1 second.
4. Breathe in as you slowly lower leg back down.
5. Repeat 10 to 15 times.
6. Repeat 10 to 15 times with other leg.
7. Repeat 10 to 15 more times with each leg.

Toe Stands

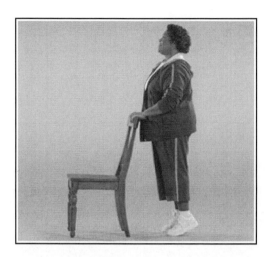

Strengthen the muscles in your calves and ankles with toe stands.

1. Stand behind a sturdy chair, feet shoulder-width apart, holding on for balance. Breathe in slowly.
2. Breathe out and slowly stand on tiptoes, as high as possible.
3. Hold position for 1 second.
4. Breathe in as you slowly lower heels to the floor.
5. Repeat 10 to 15 times.
6. Rest; then repeat 10 to 15 more times.

BALANCE EXERCISES

To get all of the benefits of physical activity, try all four types of exercise -- endurance, strength, balance, and flexibility. This section discusses balance exercises.

Important for Fall Prevention

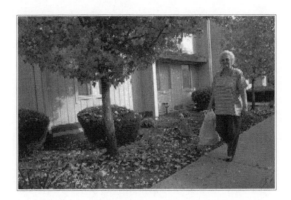

Each year, more than one-third of people age 65 or older fall. Falls and fall-related injuries, such as hip fracture, can have a serious impact on an older person's life. If you fall, it could limit your activities or make it impossible to live independently. Balance exercises, along with certain strength exercises, can help prevent falls by improving your ability to control and maintain your body's position, whether you are moving or still.

Balance Exercises to Try

The 5 exercises that follow are aimed at improving your balance and your lower body strength. They include

1. standing on one foot
2. walking heel to toe
3. balance walk

4. back leg raises
5. side leg raises

Anywhere, Anytime

You can do balance exercises almost anytime, anywhere, and as often as you like, as long as you have something sturdy nearby to hold on to if you become unsteady. In the beginning, using a chair or the wall for support will help you work on your balance safely.

Balance exercises overlap with the lower body strength exercises, which also can improve your balance. Do the strength exercises -- back leg raises, side leg raises, and hip extensions -- two or more days per week, but not on any two days in a row.

Modify as You Progress

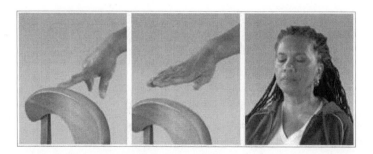

The exercises which follow can improve your balance even more if you modify them as you progress. Start by holding on to a sturdy chair for support. To challenge yourself, try holding on to the chair with only one hand; then with time, you can try holding on with only one finger, then no hands. If you are steady on your feet, try doing the exercise with your eyes closed.

Safety Tips

- Have a sturdy chair or a person nearby to hold on to if you feel unsteady.
- Talk with your doctor if you are unsure about doing a particular exercise

Standing on One Foot

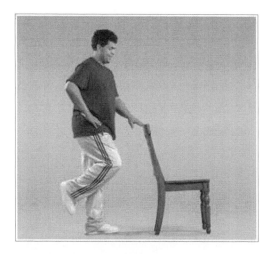

Improve your balance by standing on one foot.

1. Stand on one foot behind a sturdy chair, holding on for balance.
2. Hold position for up to 10 seconds.
3. Repeat 10 to 15 times.
4. Repeat 10 to 15 times with other leg.
5. Repeat 10 to 15 more times with each leg.

Walking Heel to Toe

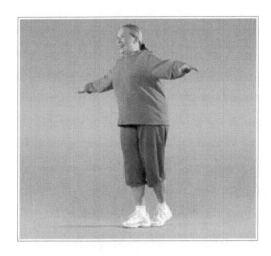

Improve your balance by walking heel to toe.

1. Position the heel of one foot just in front of the toes of the other foot. Your heel and toes should touch or almost touch.
2. Choose a spot ahead of you and focus on it to keep you steady as you walk.
3. Take a step. Put your heel just in front of the toe of your other foot.
4. Repeat for 20 steps.

Balance Walk

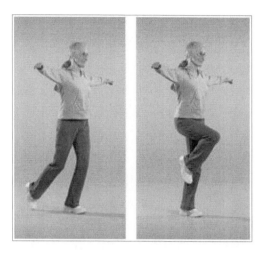

Improve your balance with the balance walk.

1. Raise arms to sides, shoulder height.
2. Choose a spot ahead of you and focus on it to keep you steady as you walk.
3. Walk in a straight line with one foot in front of the other.
4. As you walk, lift your back leg. Pause for 1 second before stepping forward.
5. Repeat for 20 steps, alternating legs.

Back Leg Raises

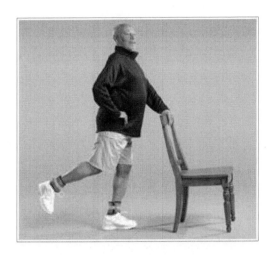

Strengthen your buttocks and lower back with back leg raises.

1. Stand behind a sturdy chair, holding on for balance. Breathe in slowly.
2. Breathe out and slowly lift one leg straight back without bending your knee or pointing your toes. Try not to lean forward. The leg you are standing on should be slightly bent.
3. Hold position for 1 second.
4. Breathe in as you slowly lower your leg.
5. Repeat 10 to 15 times.
6. Repeat 10 to 15 times with other leg.
7. Repeat 10 to 15 more times with each leg.

Side Leg Raises

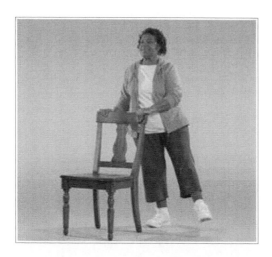

Strengthen your hips, thighs, and buttocks with side leg raises.

1. Stand behind a sturdy chair with feet slightly apart, holding on for balance. Breathe in slowly.
2. Breathe out and slowly lift one leg out to the side. Keep your back straight and your toes facing forward. The leg you are standing on should be slightly bent.
3. Hold position for 1 second.
4. Breathe in as you slowly lower your leg.
5. Repeat 10 to 15 times.
6. Repeat 10 to 15 times with other leg.
7. Repeat 10 to 15 more times with each leg.

FLEXIBILITY EXERCISES

To get all of the benefits of physical activity, try all four types of exercise -- endurance, strength, balance, and flexibility. This section discusses flexibility exercises.

More Freedom of Movement

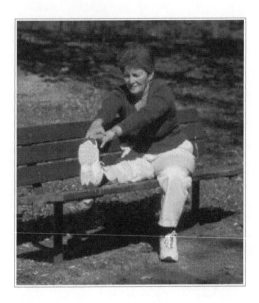

Stretching, or flexibility, exercises are an important part of your physical activity program. They give you more freedom of movement for your physical activities and for everyday activities such as getting dressed and reaching objects on a shelf. Stretching exercises can improve your flexibility but will not improve your endurance or strength.

Flexibility Exercises to Try

The 12 flexibility exercises which follow are:

1. neck stretch
2. shoulder stretch
3. shoulder and upper arm raise
4. upper body stretch
5. chest stretch
6. back stretch
7. ankle stretch
8. back of leg stretch
9. thigh stretch
10. hip stretch
11. lower back stretch
12. calf stretch

How Much Stretching Should I Do?

Do each stretching exercise 3 to 5 times at each session. Slowly stretch into the desired position, as far as possible without pain, and hold the stretch for 10 to 30 seconds. Relax, breathe, then repeat, trying to stretch farther.

You can progress in your stretching exercises. For example, as you become more flexible, try reaching farther, but not so far that it hurts.

Safety Tips

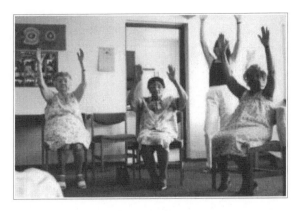

- Talk with your doctor if you are unsure about a particular exercise. For example, if you've had hip or back surgery, talk with your doctor before doing lower body exercises.
- Always warm up before stretching exercises and stretch after endurance or strength exercises. If you are doing only stretching exercises, warm up with a few minutes of easy walking first. Stretching your muscles before they are warmed up may result in injury.
- Always remember to breathe normally while holding a stretch.
- Stretching may feel slightly uncomfortable; for example, a mild pulling feeling is normal.
- You are stretching too far if you feel sharp or stabbing pain, or joint pain -- while doing the stretch or even the next day. Reduce the stretch so that it doesn't hurt.
- Never "bounce" into a stretch. Make slow, steady movements instead. Jerking into position can cause muscles to tighten, possibly causing injury.
- Avoid "locking" your joints. Straighten your arms and legs when you stretch them, but don't hold them tightly in a

straight position. Your joints should always be slightly bent while stretching.

Neck Stretch

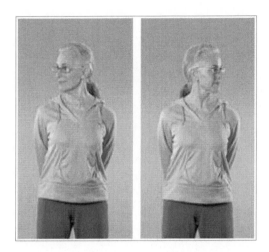

1. You can do this stretch while standing or sitting in a sturdy chair.
2. Keep your feet flat on the floor, shoulder-width apart.
3. Slowly turn your head to the right until you feel a slight stretch. Be careful not to tip or tilt your head forward or backward, but hold it in a comfortable position.
4. Hold the position for 10 to 30 seconds.
5. Turn your head to the left and hold the position for 10 to 30 seconds.
6. Repeat at least 3 to 5 times.

Shoulder Stretch

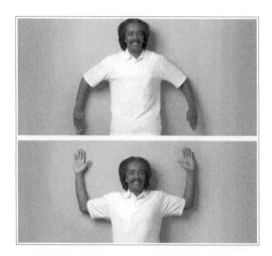

1. Stand back against a wall, feet shoulder-width apart and arms at shoulder height.
2. Bend your elbows so your fingertips point toward the ceiling and touch the wall behind you. Stop when you feel a stretch or slight discomfort, and stop immediately if you feel sharp pain.
3. Hold position for 10 to 30 seconds.
4. Let your arms slowly roll forward, remaining bent at the elbows, to point toward the floor and touch the wall again, if possible. Stop when you feel a stretch or slight discomfort.
5. Hold position for 10 to 30 seconds.
6. Alternate pointing above head, then toward hips.
7. Repeat at least 3 to 5 times.

Shoulder and Upper Arm Raise

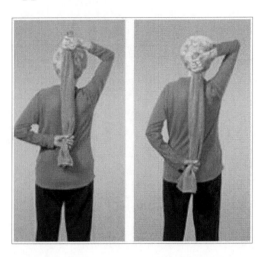

1. Stand with feet shoulder-width apart.
2. Hold one end of a towel in your right hand.
3. Raise and bend your right arm to drape the towel down your back. Keep your right arm in this position and continue holding on to the towel.
4. Reach behind your lower back and grasp the towel with your left hand.
5. To stretch your right shoulder, pull the towel down with your left hand. Stop when you feel a stretch or slight discomfort in your right shoulder.
6. Repeat at least 3 to 5 times.
7. Reverse positions, and repeat at least 3 to 5 times.

Upper Body Stretch

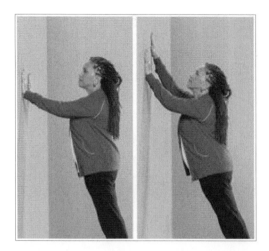

1. Stand facing a wall slightly farther than arm's length from the wall, feet shoulder-width apart.
2. Lean your body forward and put your palms flat against the wall at shoulder height and shoulder-width apart.
3. Keeping your back straight, slowly walk your hands up the wall until your arms are above your head.
4. Hold your arms overhead for about 10 to 30 seconds.
5. Slowly walk your hands back down.
6. Repeat at least 3 to 5 times.

Chest Stretch

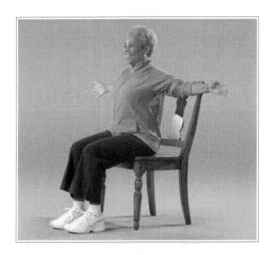

1. You can do this stretch while standing or sitting in a sturdy, armless chair.
2. Keep your feet flat on the floor, shoulder-width apart.
3. Hold arms to your sides at shoulder height, with palms facing forward.
4. Slowly move your arms back, while squeezing your shoulder blades together. Stop when you feel a stretch or slight discomfort.
5. Hold the position for 10 to 30 seconds.
6. Repeat at least 3 to 5 times.

Back Stretch

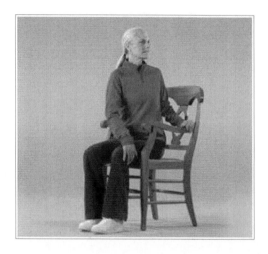

1. Sit up toward the front of a sturdy chair with armrests. Stay as straight as possible. Keep your feet flat on the floor, shoulder-width apart.
2. Slowly twist to the left from your waist without moving your hips. Turn your head to the left. Lift your left hand and hold on to the left arm of the chair. Place your right hand on the outside of your left thigh. Twist farther, if possible.
3. Hold the position for 10 to 30 seconds.
4. Slowly return to face forward.
5. Repeat on the right side.
6. Repeat at least 3 to 5 more times.

Ankle Stretch

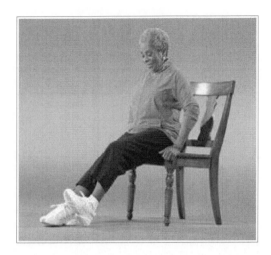

1. Sit securely toward the edge of a sturdy, armless chair.
2. Stretch your legs out in front of you.
3. With your heels on the floor, bend your ankles to point toes toward you.
4. Hold the position for 10 to 30 seconds.
5. Bend ankles to point toes away from you and hold for 10 to 30 seconds.
6. Repeat at least 3 to 5 times.

How to Get Down on the Floor

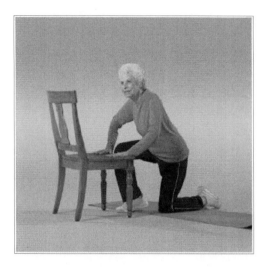

The following stretching exercises are done on the floor. To get down on the floor:

1. Stand facing the seat of a sturdy chair.
2. Put your hands on the seat, and lower yourself down on one knee.
3. Bring the other knee down.
4. Put your left hand on the floor. Leaning on your hand, slowly bring your left hip to the floor. Put your right hand on the floor next to your left hand to steady yourself, if needed.
5. You should now be sitting with your weight on your left hip.
6. Straighten your legs.
7. Bend your left elbow until your weight is resting on it. Using your right hand as needed for support, straighten your left arm. You should now be lying on your left side.
8. Roll onto your back.

If you've had hip or back surgery, talk with your doctor before using this method.

How to Get Up From the Floor

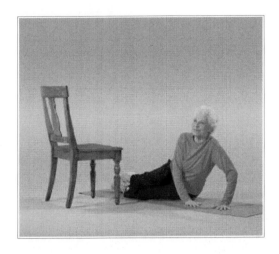

To get up from the floor:

1. Roll onto your left side.
2. Place your right hand on the floor at about the level of your ribs and use it to push your shoulders off the floor. Use your left hand to help lift you up, as needed.
3. You should now be sitting with your weight on your left hip.
4. Roll forward, onto your knees, leaning on your hands for support.
5. Reach up and lean your hands on the seat of a sturdy chair.
6. Lift one of your knees so that one leg is bent, foot flat on the floor.
7. Leaning your hands on the seat of the chair for support, rise from this position.

If you've had hip or back surgery, talk with your doctor before using this method.

Back of Leg Stretch

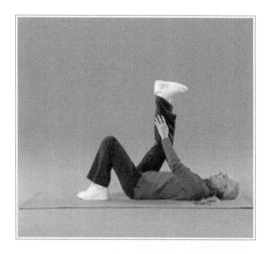

1. Lie on your back with left knee bent and left foot flat on the floor.
2. Raise right leg, keeping knee slightly bent.
3. Reach up and grasp right leg with both hands. Keep head and shoulders flat on the floor.
4. Gently pull right leg toward your body until you feel a stretch in the back of your leg.
5. Hold position for 10 to 30 seconds.
6. Repeat at least 3 to 5 times.
7. Repeat at least 3 to 5 times with left leg.

Thigh Stretch

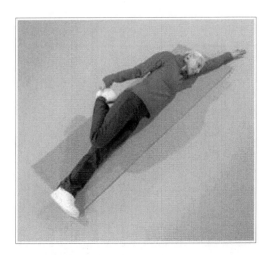

1. Lie on your side with legs straight and knees together.
2. Rest your head on your arm.
3. Bend top knee and reach back and grab the top of your foot. If you can't reach your foot, loop a resistance band, belt, or towel over your foot and hold both ends.
4. Gently pull your leg until you feel a stretch in your thigh.
5. Hold position for 10 to 30 seconds.
6. Repeat at least 3 to 5 times.
7. Repeat at least 3 to 5 times with your other leg.

Hip Stretch

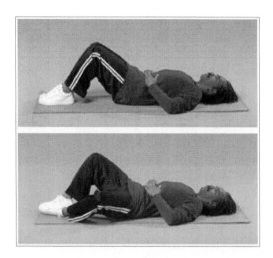

1. Lie on your back with your legs together, knees bent, and feet flat on the floor. Try to keep both shoulders on the floor throughout the stretch.
2. Slowly lower one knee as far as you comfortably can. Keep your feet close together and try not to move the other leg.
3. Hold position for 10 to 30 seconds.
4. Bring knee back up slowly.
5. Repeat at least 3 to 5 times.
6. Repeat at least 3 to 5 times with your other leg.

Lower Back Stretch

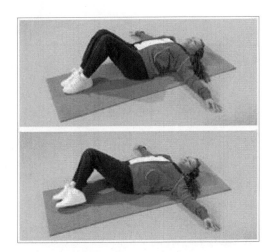

1. Lie on your back with your legs together, knees bent, and feet flat on the floor. Try to keep both arms and shoulders flat on the floor throughout the stretch.
2. Keeping knees bent and together, slowly lower both legs to one side as far as you comfortably can.
3. Hold position for 10 to 30 seconds.
4. Bring legs back up slowly and repeat toward other side.
5. Continue alternating sides for at least 3 to 5 times on each side.

Calf Stretch

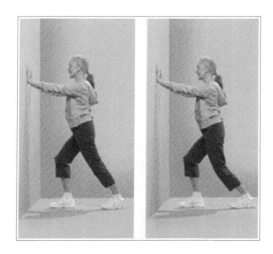

1. Stand facing a wall slightly farther than arm's length from the wall, feet shoulder-width apart.
2. Put your palms flat against the wall at shoulder height and shoulder-width apart.
3. Step forward with right leg and bend right knee. Keeping both feet flat on the floor, bend left knee slightly until you feel a stretch in your left calf muscle. It shouldn't feel uncomfortable. If you don't feel a stretch, bend your right knee until you do.
4. Hold position for 10 to 30 seconds, and then return to starting position.
5. Repeat with left leg.
6. Continue alternating legs for at least 3 to 5 times on each leg.

BIBLIOGRAPHY

National Institute on Aging. *Exercise: How to Get Started. Retrieved* February 19, 2014 from http://nihseniorhealth.gov/exerciseandphysicalactivityhowtogetstarted/safetyfirst/01.html

National Institute on Aging. *Exercise: Exercises to Try*. February 19, 2014 from http://nihseniorhealth.gov/exerciseandphysicalactivityexercisestotry/enduranceexercises/01.html

Printed in Great Britain
by Amazon.co.uk, Ltd.,
Marston Gate.